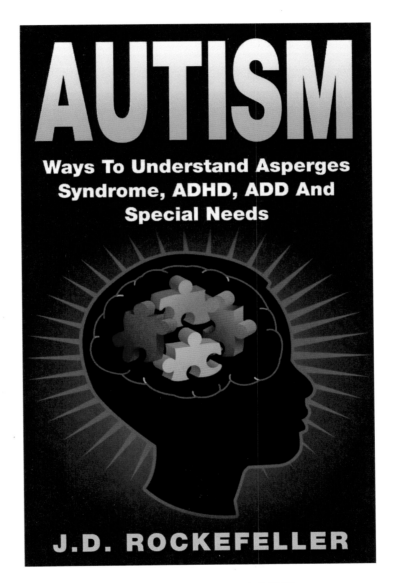

J.D.ROCKEFELLER

Table of Contents

Introduction

Autism is defined as neuro-developmental disorder that is characterized by repetitive and restricted behavior, verbal and non-verbal communication and impaired social interaction. Signs are normally noted during the first two years of their children being born. Signs normally develop gradually over time, though certain children with autism may reach their developmental achievements at normal pace and regress. The entire diagnostic criteria require that symptoms become evident during early childhood, normally within the first three years of birth.

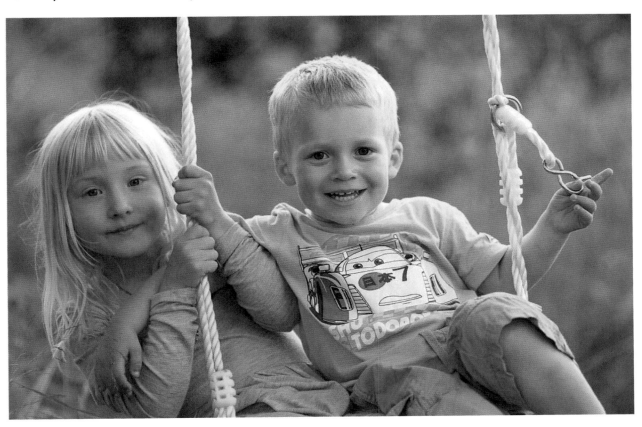

Although autism is a highly heritable condition, research studies indicate genetic and environmental factors to be the main causes. In certain cases, although rare, autism is largely associated with elements that cause birth defects. There is a lot of controversy that surrounds different other suggested environmental causes, for instance, the hypotheses on vaccine have been unproven. Autism has an effect on the way in which the brain processes information by changing the manner nerve cells and synapses organize and connect; how this happens is not really understood. It's among the three disorders of the autism spectrum, with the other two being Asperger syndrome and pervasive developmental disorder (PDD). Asperger syndrome defines a delay in language and cognitive development and PDD is not really specified but diagnosed when a complete set of criteria for Asperger syndrome or autism are not met.

Behavioral interventions or early speech can enable children with autism to gain self-care, communication, and social skills. While there isn't a known cure for the condition, there have been some reported cases about children who've recovered. A few children with autism get to live independently after they reach adulthood, although some go on to become successful. In recent times, a new autistic culture has become advent, with some people searching for a cure and some believing that the condition should be accepted and not treated like a disorder.

Based on data from 2010, the number of people with autism was estimated to be about 1-2 for every 1,000 people globally. The condition is also 4-5 times more likely to develop among boys than girls. An estimated 1.7 percent of children in the U.S. are diagnosed with the condition, and as of 2014 there had been a 30 percent increase from 1 in 88 in 2012. Autism among adults in the United Kingdom is 1.1 percent. The number of new cases has increased dramatically from the 1980s, largely because of changes in government-subsidized financial incentives and diagnostic practice for named diagnoses, but the question of whether the actual rates have risen remains unresolved.

Asperger Syndrome: Definition and Symptoms

Asperger syndrome is defined as a developmental disorder which makes it extremely difficult to socially interact with others. You child may experience difficulty in making friends because of their social awkwardness.

Individuals with Asperger syndrome also exhibit certain attributes of autism. For instance, they may exhibit poor interaction skills, prefer routine things and not been keen on change. But different to people with autism, children who suffer from Asperger syndrome normally begin talking before they reach the age of 2, a time when speech develops among infants.

When someone has Asperger syndrome, it's generally a lifetime condition, but the symptoms may improve over time. Adults suffering from this condition can learn with time how to understand their own strengths and weaknesses. And better yet even improve their social interaction skills.

Both autism and Asperger syndrome are classified as autism spectrum disorders and previously called pervasive developmental disorders. At times, you may hear people use ASD to refer to Asperger syndrome.

The main causes of Asperger syndrome are not known as well as how to prevent it from occurring. The condition is largely heritable and runs in families. Researchers are still conducting studies to find out the genetic causes of Asperger syndrome. The condition also tends to affect more males than their female counterparts.

The condition is normally noticed around the ages of 3 or beyond. Symptoms vary widely, and for that no children will exhibit the same attributes. Children with Asperger syndrome:

• Experience difficulty relating to other people. It does not mean that they keep away from social interaction, but rather they don't have the skills and instincts to enable them share their thoughts and feelings as well as take note of others' feelings.

• Prefer their fixed routines and change is very hard for them.

• May be uncomfortable around loud noises, textures, strong tastes or lights

• May not understand social norms or recognize verbal and non-verbal cues. For instance, they might stare at others, not know the meaning of personal space or eye contact.

• May have flat and difficult to understand speech because it lacks accent, pitch, and tone. Or they may actually have some formal way of speaking that's just too developed for their age.

• May have bad handwriting or experience difficulty with other motorized skills like riding a bicycle.

• May lack some level of personal coordination; have unorthodox body postures, gestures, facial expressions or just be clumsy.

- May have a limited number of interests or may intensely focus on limited things. For instance, they may exhibit a usual interest in snakes and scorpions or tree names or may actually draw detailed pictures.

Tests and Exams

Asperger syndrome is classified as a developmental condition which makes people experience difficulty in understanding social interaction. A proper diagnosis will include input from doctors, teachers and parents as well as other caregivers who've observed or know the child. Asperger syndrome can be diagnosed when a specific criteria is met. They include:

- Unusual behavior, activities, and interests

- Poor social interaction

- No delay in the development of language

- No delay in interest about the environment and self-help skills

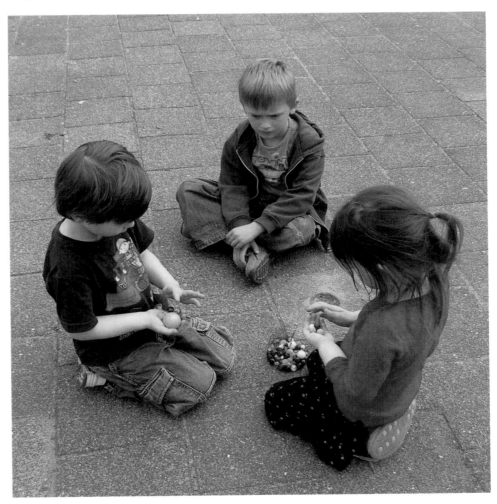

A doctor will look into your medical history by asking a number of questions about how your child is developing, including information about language and motor development, social interactions and areas of specific interest. The doctor will also need information relating to the parent's pregnancy as well as the family's medical history.

Testing may help you doctor determine whether your child's condition is related to Asperger syndrome. Your care provider will refer your child to a specialist for exams and tests, including:

• Communication assessment. Formal language and speech are evaluated. Tests are performed on children to determine how they use and understand language to communicate their ideas. The doctor will also perform tests for understanding non-verbal and non-literal forms of language skills and communication, like understanding metaphor or humor. Your doctor will listen to your child's volume of voice, pitch and stress.

• Psychological assessment. Style of learning and intellectual function are evaluated. Intelligence quotient (IQ) and motor skill tests are quite common. Other tests like personality assessment tests can also be done.

• Psychiatric examination. The doctor may also examine your child's peer and family relationships, responses to different situations as well as the ability to understand feelings of other forms of indirect communication like sarcasm and teasing. Your doctor may also be keen on observing your child at school or at home. He or she may certain conditions like depression and anxiety, which are commonly associated with people suffering from Asperger Syndrome.

How Asperger Syndrome is Diagnosed?

If there are any symptoms, your doctor will do an evaluation by conducting a thorough medical history and neurological and physical exam. Many people with Asperger syndrome experience coordination issues, dyspraxia and low muscle tone. While there are no tests to determine Asperger syndrome, doctors use different tests like blood tests and x-rays to find out if there are other disorders of physical issues causing the symptoms.

If physical disorder isn't found, your child may then be referred to some specialist who deals with childhood development disorders like a psychologist, adolescent and child psychiatrist, developmental-behavioral pediatrician, pediatric neurologist or some other health care professional who's trained to treat Asperger syndrome. The doctor will be able to diagnose the child's development, as well as observe the child's behavior and speech, including how they play and the manner in which they socially interact with other people. The doctor will normally need input from the child's teachers, parents, and any other adults familiar with the symptoms.

How Asperger Syndrome is Treated?

Asperger Syndrome currently doesn't have a cure, but certain therapies may reduce unwanted behaviors and improve functioning. Treatment of the syndrome will generally include a combination of:

- Behavior modification: This will include using certain strategies that support positive behavior as well as reduce problem behaviors.

- Special education.This involves developing education that's structured to suit the child's individual educational needs.

- Physical, speech and or occupational therapy: Such therapies are developed to enhance a child's functional ability.

- Social skills therapies: Make a trip to a speech pathologist, social worker, counselor or psychologist, these therapies offer invaluable ways to improve social skills as well as the ability to interpret verbal and nonverbal cues which often lack in people with Asperger syndrome.

Medications: There are currently no medications used to treat Asperger syndrome, but certain drugs may be used to reduce symptoms like depression, anxiety, obsessive-compulsive behavior and hyperactivity.

ADHD and ADD: Definition and Types

Overview of ADHD

Attention deficit hyperactivity disorder also referred to as (ADHD) as well as attention deficit disorder, also referred to as (ADD) exhibit symptoms that can start in childhood and go into adulthood. Both ADHD and ADD symptoms, like inattentiveness, impulsiveness, and hyperactivity, can cause serious problems at work, school, home and or in relationships.

Unlike cancer or a broken bone, ADHD also known as ADD doesn't exhibit physical signs that can be detected by lab or blood tests. Typical symptoms of ADHD often overlap those of other psychological and physical disorders. Causes of the condition are not known, but doctors can diagnose ADHD and effectively treat it. There are many resources available to support and help families manage ADHD behaviors if they occur.

What Are The Types of ADHD

The three types of ADHD are:

1.   Inattentive

Normally referred to when the term ADD is used. This defines a person who shows symptoms of inattention, meaning they can be easily distracted, but not impulsive or hyperactive.

2.   Hyperactive-Impulsive

A type that normally takes place after a person shows symptoms of impulsivity and hyperactivity and not inattention.

3.   Combined

Occurs when a person exhibits symptoms of hyperactivity, impulsivity, and inattention

Symptoms of ADHD

Any child can fidget and have trouble in paying attention. A child, however with ADHD will have such symptoms to such an extent that they become distractions at home or at school.

The three major symptoms are:

•   Inattention

•   Impulsiveness

•   Hyperactivity

Each of these symptoms comes with certain criteria a child needs to meet to be diagnosed. The criteria required for proper diagnosis will vary according to age and gender. Children who 16 and above need to exhibit 6 or more symptoms, and those over 17 need just 5.

Symptoms need to be prevalent for a period no less than 6 months and should inappropriate with the child's developmental stage.

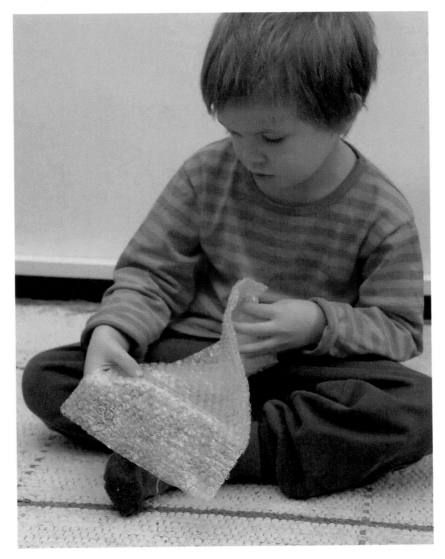

"Bubble wrap play" by Miika Silfverberg (MiikaS) from Vantaa, Finland - Flickr. Licensed under CC BY-SA 2.0 via Wikimedia Commons - https://commons.wikimedia.org/wiki/File:Bubble_wrap_play.jpg#/media/File:Bubble_wrap_play.jpg

Inattention

Trouble focusing or inattention is another ADHD symptom. Any child can be diagnosed as inattentive if he or she is:

- Easily distracted

- Forgetful, even for daily activities

- Experiencing difficulty in being attentive to activities and tasks

- Fails to bear close attention to different details of school work and other activities, like making random and careless mistakes

- Ignores speakers, even when directly spoken to

- Doesn't follow instructions, loses focus on activities, fails to complete chores or homework and is easily sidetracked

- Avoids and dislikes tasks requiring prolonged periods of mental work, like homework

- Has trouble being organized

- Constantly loses important things necessary for activities and tasks like books, wallet, keys, calculator, pencil cases and so on.

Hyperactivity and Impulsivity

Any child can be hyperactive and or impulsive if he or she:

- Always appears to be on the move

- Talks excessively

- Have extreme difficulty in waiting for their turn

- Gets up from their seat when they are expected to be seated

- Fidgets, taps their hands and feet or squirms when seating

- Climbs and runs around in appropriate situations

- Cannot play quietly or participate in recreational activities

- Shouts out answers even before the question is finished

- Interrupts and intrudes constantly

More Criteria

In addition to symptoms of impulsivity, hyperactivity and attention, children or adults should also meet the following criteria:

- Exhibit a number of symptoms before they reach the age of 12

- Display symptoms in different settings like at home, school, with friends and during other activities

- Symptoms can't be explained by other conditions like anxiety, psychotic and mood disorders

- Shows evidence that symptoms interfere with functionality at work, school or have an impact on how they socialize with other peers.

Adult

If an adult has ADHD, then it's likely that they've had the condition since childhood, but without being diagnosed until later on in their life. Evaluation normally occurs after a friend, family member, co-worker or some other close person observes the problems in relationships or at work.

Diagnoses of adults can be done using any of the subtypes of ADHD. Symptoms of ADHD in adults are normally different to those of children because of the maturity adults possess as well as the different physical attributes between children and adults.

Severity

Symptoms can vary from mild to severe largely depending on the person's environment and physiology. Some individuals may experience mild hyperactivity or inattentiveness when they do tasks they don't love but have the ability to focus more on those tasks they love. Some may experience severe symptoms, and these may impact negatively at work, in social setups and in school.

Symptoms tend to be severe non-structured group situations, for instance, on playgrounds than in structured setups were rewards are presented like in classrooms. Other conditions like anxiety, a learning disability or depression many worsen symptoms. Certain individuals report that their symptoms dissipate as they grow older. For instance, an adult diagnosed with ADHD who was hyperactive during childhood may discover that he or she is now able to curb their impulsivity.

Outlook

The fortunate thing is that you are now closer to discovering the appropriate treatment by determining the kind of ADD you suffer from and its level of severity. Make sure you discuss all the symptoms you experience with your doctor to help in being accurately diagnosed, and this will be your first step to receiving the right treatment.

Dealing with People with ADHD

Dealing with people who have ADHD is no easy feat. It can be very difficult to help a family member or friend diagnosed with ADHD, although the chances are that it's even much harder for them to cope with the condition. With that being the case, stick to it and employ some useful tips to help manage their symptoms.

This may help if:

- You need to help someone with ADHD

- You have a friend or family member with ADHD

- You have ADHD and it's hard on the patient

Understanding ADHD

ADHD is defined as a behavioral disorder where a person experiences difficulty in focusing on their tasks and activities. If you have a friend or family member who's got ADHD, it is very important to know that they won't always relate to different people the same. They will normally struggle with symptoms like:

- Failure to pay attention or remain focused

- Being impatient

- Not follow instructions

- Lose things and or be forgetful

- Make careless mistakes at work or school

- Fail to follow up on instructions or complete tasks

- Get easily distracted

- Easily lose attention when some are speaking to them

- Not able to remain sitting still

- Talk a lot

- Not able to quietly do things

- Interrupt and butt into people's conversations

- Have trouble relating to people's points of view and emotions

Such attributes can make it very difficult for anyone to nurture a friendship the way want to.

For this reason, it is important that you stand by your friends' or family member's side, and don't take things personally if they are not always in the same bracket as you.

How you can help

• Understand and recognize that the condition is beyond their control: If some constantly exhibit the previously mentioned symptoms, you may find yourself increasingly getting frustrated. Should this happen, just tell yourself that it wasn't their choice to be like that. It may test your patience to the limit, but keep in mind that you'll be doing the best thing for them.

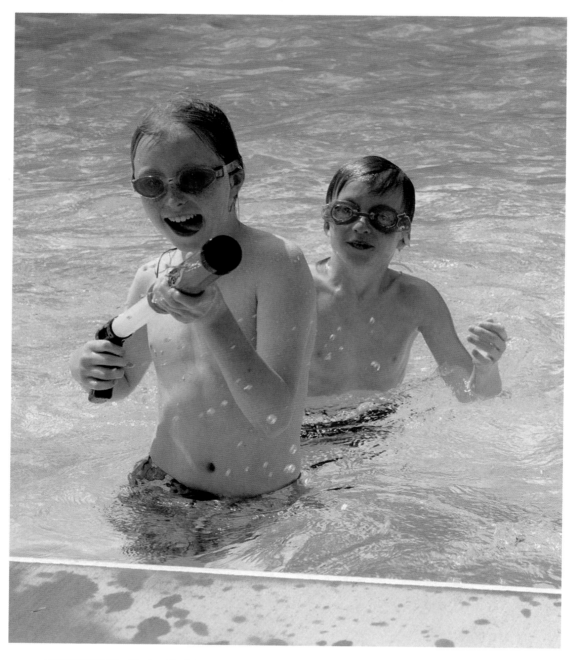

• Be forgiving: We do stuff up from time to time, but you may find your friend or family member starting to make frequent mistakes. Be forgiving even if you believe that they are doing it deliberately, being careless or lazy.

• Get as much information: Find out as much information as possible about ADHD as it may help you understand what they are experiencing.

• Encourage them to take their medication: Encourage them to stick with their medication and treatment plan. Getting the right medication be a bit tricky sometimes, and frustrating. If they get discouraged, encourage them to take their medication and see a doctor. Stopping abruptly on medication can be dangerous.

Conclusion

The major objectives when treating a child with autism is to reduce family distress and associated deficits and to enhance functional independence and quality of life. There isn't a single treatment that's best and the treatment will normally be tailored to suit the child's individual needs. The educational system and the family provide most resources for the treatment.

Research studies on interventions have drawn methodological issues that have hindered definitive conclusions on efficacy. While numerous psychosocial interventions have shown some positive evidence which suggests that even some form of treatment is much better than no treatment, the quality of the methodological approach, as well as the systematic reviews of the studies, has been generally poor, clinical results have been tentative at most with little evidence to indicate the effectiveness of different treatment options.

OTHER BOOKS BY J.D.ROCKEFELLER

If you liked this book then you might enjoy other J.D. Rockefeller titles listed below. Also, stay tuned for more exciting new titles that will be released soon by subscribing to J.D. Rockefeller's Newsletter!

You may also like other books from the Author:

"The Paleo Diet: A Beginner's Guide"

"Understanding Candida: Causes, Treatment and Cure"

"How to Stop Hair Loss and Regrow It Naturally Without Compromising on Safety"

"Container Gardening for Beginners"

"Chakras for Beginners: How to balance chakras, strengthen aura, and radiate energy"

"Bikram Yoga Poses and their Benefits"

"How to Get Rid of Cellulite"

"How to Declutter and Organize your House in 30 Minutes: Great Organizing Tips"

"Minimalist Living: How To Declutter, Simplify And Organize Your Life"

"Chakras Easy Guide for Beginners: Chakra Meditation, Understanding and Balancing the 7 Chakras"

"Auras: How to See and Read Auras"

"Greatest Motivational and Inspirational Quotes on Life, Love and Happiness"

"Simple guide to Feminization by Mistress Dede"

"Essential Oils Guide: How to Use Aromatherapy and Essential Oils"

"The Green Smoothie Recipe Diet: How to Cleanse and Detox and Lose up to 15 Pounds in 10 Days!"

"Juicing Recipes for Health and Weight Loss: How to Lose Weight with the Juicing Diet"

"The Introvert Personality: The Advantage of Introverts in an Extrovert World"

"The Coffee Enema Book"

"Chakra Healing Test: Which Chakras Do You Need to Balance"

SPECIAL FACEBOOK GROUP

Come join our Facebook group just for readers like you who want to read informative, interesting, practical books to enhance everyday life. In this group we'll be sharing our tips and knowledge with each other, so that we can all contribute to enriching and empowering our lives.

This is also a fantastic group for finding inspiration and new ideas! Imagine the impact you could have if you had hundreds of other people from all over the world collaborating with you on how to make your life better.

It's also a great place to get any life questions or special interest questions you have answered.

Come join us here on Facebook: Fountain of Knowledge Books

CONNECT WITH J.D.ROCKEFELLER

Thank you so much for taking the time to read this book. If you have questions, feel free to contact me directly at ebook_downloads@yahoo.com

You can follow me on Twitter: @E_bookDownload

And connect with me on Facebook: The Fountain of Knowledge Books

Visit my blog at: www.MyFreeEbookDownload.com

I wish you all the best of health, happiness and inspiration!

Cheers,

J.D. Rockefeller

ABOUT THE AUTHOR

J.D.ROCKEFELLER is an internationally renowned author with a simple, yet engaging writing style. An avid world traveler and wine connoisseur, he enjoys looking at the world through a writer's lens and putting his thoughts to paper everywhere he goes.

We invite you to stay tuned for many of his upcoming writings by visiting www.myfreeebookdownload.com

Message from the Author:

"It is my absolute pleasure to connect with you, my readers, on topics that you enjoy and want to learn more about. As a full-time writer, it is my passion to learn about and research exciting subjects, as well as bring you practical knowledge that may help you to enhance your daily life.

I sincerely hope that you will accompany me on this beautiful journey of knowledge which will not only entertain you but will also richly broaden your intellectual horizons.

Please know that one of my true passions is to interact with my readers and to learn what they like reading about, as well as get their feedback on my work. So, feel free to reach out to me at any time. I am here for you and because of you: my readers who have followed me and continue to share my work year after year." Learn more at: www.myfreeebookdownload.com

ONE LAST THING...

Thank you for reading this book! If you enjoyed it or found it helpful, I would be very grateful if you would post a short review on Amazon. Your great support makes a tremendous difference, and I personally read all the reviews so I can get your feedback and continue to improve this book.

Thank you very much for your support!

AUTISM

Ways To Understand Asperges Syndrome, ADHD, ADD And Special Needs

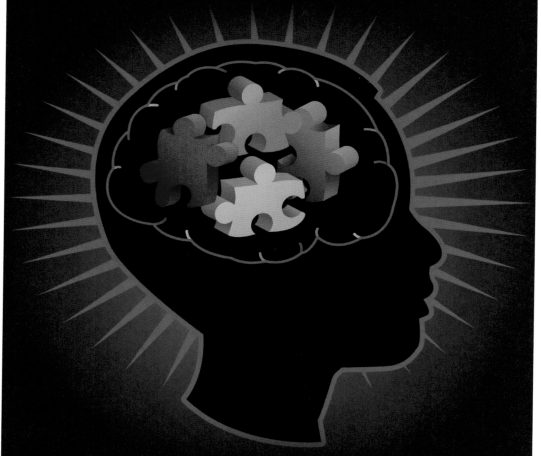

J.D. ROCKEFELLER

Printed in Great Britain
by Amazon